Lucinda 2.0

Luci Jenkin

DEDICATION

This story is written for L, H and J. I really couldn't have got through the last 18 months without your help and support.

And to BL. I know I am not allowed to thank you, so perhaps this will show you how much I appreciate all that you have done.

CONTENTS

ACKNOWLEDGMENTS

Thank you to all my friends and family who have been such a support to me throughout this journey. I really wouldn't have made the recovery I have without you.

PREFACE

This is my story. This is the journey from the diagnosis of my brain tumour, to trying to accept the new me. It is my version of what has happened, told from my perspective. If you want to know what L thought of things, you will need to ask him and/or get him to tell his own story.

Some parts of this will be hard to read - they might be graphic, not very pleasant or just not what people who are on the journey with me would like to read. However, in order for it to be of some use to others who may be on a similar path, I feel all those details need to be put in.

At the back of this story is a by no means exhaustive list of people to thank. If I've missed you out, I'm very sorry

- blame the tumour!

PART 1

2018 – The Year of Survival

My story begins at the end of August, 2018. I had been having a few odd symptoms for several months. My balance was a bit off - when on a school residential, I got up one morning and wobbled into the wall. "Been on the drink already have you?" my roommate asked. (I put this down to getting up too quickly and lack of sleep.) I had tingly extremities - bad circulation? Tingly and numb areas on my face? This one was not so easy to explain. I phoned my GP for an appointment. The first time, I was told to phone back in a few weeks when there were more doctors available. The second time, I was told a doctor would phone me back later that day. This happened and I was asked to go in for an appointment in a couple of days. I then got a call asking me to come in later that day. A variety of tests were done on me by my GP and I was told "nothing to worry about but I will send you for a CT scan, just to be sure"

On 7th September, the radiology department at my local hospital, The Alexandra, rang to say they had a cancellation for 8:30 the following morning (a Saturday) if I could make it.

I set off assuming I be back home sitting on the sofa with my son (J) in less than an hour, enjoying a cuppa. I came out of my scan and the technician told me to come back at 9:00 as the radiologist needed to speak to me. I knew this meant something wasn't quite right but was not overly worried. I decided to go to the nearby Tesco to get the ingredients my daughter (H) needed for her cooking extravaganza for the upcoming cycle race our club was hosting.

At 9:00 I was back in the radiology department. The radiographer asked me in and told me they had found something in my scan. I was to go to the next door A&E department straight away. I phoned my husband (L) who was on his way to go sailing with J. They turned around. H rang to find out where I was. She was slightly alarmed to find out I was at hospital. Some friends (B&M) were then called upon to be with the children while L came to the hospital to be with me while we tried to work out what was going on.

I remember a very frustrating day. I was told I had a lesion (or tumour or growth or mass depending on who I spoke to). It would require treatment. The best place for this was at University Hospital, Coventry and Warwick (UHCW) in another county about 50 minutes away. I needed to wait for a bed to become available. No, I couldn't wait at home. No reason was given. The nurses just kept saying they were told I had to stay where I was. Finally a bed was free. But we needed to wait for an ambulance. No, my husband couldn't drive me there. What was going on? Nobody would answer any questions. A friend, who was a nurse working in A&E kept checking in on me. But she wouldn't tell me anything either, only that the hospital I was going to was the best place to be.

The children arrived during the morning. They were tearful. We shared lots of hugs but we couldn't tell them anything. L and I made a promise to them at that point. We would keep no secrets from them. At the time they were 15 and 11. We kept to our promise - although sometimes we didn't tell them everything - particularly to J The family went home at some point, partly to give them a break and partly to go and put together a bag for me. I knew I would be in hospital for a few days.

While waiting for an ambulance, I heard the on-duty nurse talking on the phone to my new hospital. It was then I heard the size of the growth/mass/tumour/lesion. "It is about 8-9 cm in diameter" I heard. Yikes! That didn't sound too good. There were a lot of other words used, some of which I understood, some I didn't. I was beginning to get the idea that this was quite serious. Eventually, an ambulance was free to take me to my new home. L was able to follow in the car but not able to come with me. Another friend (J) was called in to come and sit with the children. B & M had been at our house for most of the day. Not quite the Saturday they had planned....

I was taken up the motorway with lights flashing and sirens wailing. Quite exciting really (but why all the fuss??) I arrived at the hospital at about 10:00p.m. I think. I was booked in and taken to my new "bedroom" which I shared with 5 other ladies. A doctor came to take some bloods. This is a job best left to the phlebotomists.... I was left with an amazing bruise and some bloods that needed taking in the morning! I was finally allowed to get some sleep - by this time it was about one in the morning. Little did I know that this building would be my home for the next 3 months….!

The next few days are a bit of a blur - I know things that happened, but not necessarily in what order. On Sunday, I was visited by a consultant. He said I had a large tumour, in a difficult place. More would be known after an MRI scan which would hopefully take place on the Monday.

L and the children went to help out at the aforementioned cycle race. We wanted life to continue to be as normal for them as possible and this event was one that we had all been looking forward to. News of my predicament spread fairly quickly. One of the main organisers of the day was my friend who had been with the children all day Saturday. It only took a few people asking where I was for her to take them aside and tell them - as much for her to be able to talk about it, as for others to learn. It was also helpful for some key people to know in case either of the children or L were a bit out of sorts.

I also remember phoning my boss while hanging out of a window (the phone reception at the hospital was rubbish but the wi-fi surprisingly good as I found out.) Very soon communications were made by email (or skype/whatsapp). I told her I had a brain tumour which would need removing with an operation but I expected to be back at work in a week or two.

The most difficult part of the day came in the evening when the family came to visit. We still had to let my parents know. There followed lots of discussion about how to let them know. They would be shocked, have questions and there would probably be tears. We decided to phone my brother to let him know the news and ask him to then tell my parents. We would then phone them a few minutes later. The hope was that at least some of the shock would have worn off by then. I'm not sure if it worked - you would have to ask them. There then followed a difficult conversation - mostly because we still knew very little about what was going on ourselves.

On Monday, I was sent for my first MRI (with contrast). While a CT scan gives a general picture of what is going on (there was a tumour within my skull), an MRI gives a more detailed picture of exactly where it spreads to and how big it is. Adding contrast in shows the blood vessels around it. Although I could walk, I was taken down in a wheelchair by some lovely porters. Once I was in the MRI room, I had to have a venflon put in so that they could put the contrast in at a certain point during the scan. This is a job normally done up on the ward. While I couldn't really feel the needle going into my arm, I could certainly feel the pool of blood growing underneath it! Once that was all sorted (!), I was told what would happen in the MRI - lots of loud whirring, some clunking and then, when the dye went in, it would feel like I had wet myself. I didn't really understand what that meant, but thought it would just feel a little odd. Suffice to say, it really does feel like you have wet yourself - warm and wet down the insides of your legs. You will be pleased to know that all clothing remained dry - but it was a very odd feeling (and the description is very accurate)!!

Then a consultant came to see me to explain the results of the MRI. The tumour was a very large meningioma (about 10cm in diameter (the size of a grapefruit) and in a very tricky position. It was at the place where my skull and spinal column meet. There were blood vessels surrounding it and lots of nerves involved. My consultant said he was passing me over to another consultant, Mr Radu Beltechi. He was the best at removing my sort of tumour and had lots of experience with tricky tumours. That was the good news. The bad news was that Mr Beltechi was away on a conference for the next week so my operation would have to wait.

I asked if I could go home. The answer was an emphatic no. It was now that I realised why I had not been able to go home on the Saturday. My tumour position and size was explained to me like this... "Imagine your skull is a sink. It is filled with spinal fluid. Your tumour is acting like a plug, stopping the fluid draining down the spinal column - as it should do. Your fluid is very, very near the overflow. If the fluid starts going through the overflow, the results could be catastrophic. You will need surgery immediately." While I was allowed out of the ward, pre-op, I was not to be on my own in case "the sink overflowed". So now I had some answers. And while I felt absolutely fine, I realised that I was in quite a serious situation.

So the next 10 or so days were quite odd. I was in hospital, having all the hospital checks, but felt absolutely fine. I spent the rest of the first week practically "putting my house in order". I had a governors meeting at a local school for which I was (and still am) Chair of governors. A document I wanted to present was finished off and sent to the Vice-Chair - along with a request that he take over as Chair for the foreseeable future. As we had just appointed a new Headteacher, and I was hoping to support his induction, not being around was something I felt particularly bad about. I made sure my husband had the passwords to the accounts for the children so he could top up their meal credits etc. I made sure that the cycling bag that I took each week to the youth coaching sessions was located and passed on to someone who could run them. And sorting out lifts to and from school for the children? L sorted those out in the main, but I had to confirm a few bits and pieces. I spun many plates, pre op, and it turns out most of them could carry on spinning in my absence.

The first half of the second week was spent mentally "putting my house in order". I always thought I would come out the other side of my operation - despite the risks. So I spent the days appreciating my four walls, looking at the hedge I could see from my bed and watching it change ever so slowly each day. I decided I no longer wanted to be on one committee, and I would slowly pull back from another activity but knew that I really enjoyed governance and that would be a priority to return to. From listening to other ladies experiences with meningiomas, I thought I would be out of action for a few weeks while I got over the surgery but really, meningiomas were the best of the types of brain tumour to get (they are classified as a grade 1 tumour - benign and very, very unlikely to spread to other parts of the body - although that can only be confirmed once the tumour is taken out and analysed).

I had various experiences over the 10 days. One of the most memorable is how quickly you get to know your fellow patients - and how quickly bed occupants change. In my first 2 weeks in hospital, I saw 24 different occupants of the five beds in my bay. While people are in, you share so much of your experience with other people - from diagnosis to departure. From how often people need bed pans (if they are capable of asking for them) to when they open their bowels. One of the questions you are asked very regularly by the nurses or health care assistants (HCAs) is if you have opened your bowels today. And what number was it? This number refers to the number your poo is on the Bristol Stool Scale. I shall leave you to research this at your will.....

I remember talking to a lady for over 3 hours one night when neither of us could sleep. We covered all sorts of topics and in another time, may have become good friends. She left the next day, and that was that. I struck up a good relationship with another lady in the bed opposite mine. We chatted a lot, and I chatted to her family a fair bit. Her tumour was unfortunately a grade 3. She had already had cancer so this was a return. Although they could take out a lot of her tumour, her outcome was not likely to be as positive as mine. She was out of the ward when I went to have my op. I never saw her again as she was discharged by the time I came back.

But we also shared moments of great joy as women came in, had their tumours removed and were sent home in a few days. Or came in with neurological symptoms, had them diagnosed and were sent home on medication. But over those two or three days, we had all shared an intense relationship.

I remember a very sad story. One of the ladies in our bay was Polish. She was a very lively lady and we managed to communicate with her with gestures, smiles and a few words. She had had a brain tumour removed. One day a large number of people came to sit by her bed. Her brother-in-law and his wife (her husband was a shift worker and at work), a nurse, a translator and a Macmillan nurse. The blue curtains were drawn in an attempt to give her some privacy. (The blue curtains give a semblance of privacy, and although you cannot see what is going on behind them, you can pretty much hear everything).We all listened as our poor friend was given the news that her brain tumour, although it had been removed, had already metastasised to her lungs and liver. She was likely to be dead by Christmas. Once the curtains were drawn back and all the visitors had left, we tried to sympathise with her. But what could we say? She told us that it would be ok and she was going to really enjoy her last days and make the most of them. What an amazing lady.

I was very entertained by one experience I had. One morning 3 gentlemen came into the bay. It wasn't visiting time. Who were they? My bed was the first one they came to. "Hello. We are from hospital radio. We would like to play a request for you. What would you like us to play?" Now this posed a problem for me. Anyone who knows me knows that I love singing and listening to music. I sing in a choir too. So asking for a song to play was pretty difficult. I summarised my problem for them - there are so many songs I could request. How do I choose? "Pick anything" they said. "So far this morning, we have had requests as different as Mozart to The Beatles, and yesterday we even had a request for The Gas Man Cometh by a duo called

Flanders and Swann". Now this gave me an idea. "I love Flanders and Swann" I replied to a slightly surprised trio. (For those of you who don't know, Flanders and Swann did an act in the 1960's combining very clever songs with jokes and talking. Their most famous numbers include the Hippopotamus song and A Transport of Delight - about London buses.) "Could you play An Ill Wind by Flanders and Swann?" I asked. "Which one is that?" one of them replied. "The one about Mozart's horn concerto" I said. "Right - we will play that on our show tonight. Who would you like to dedicate it to?" So, if there was a random song about a horn concerto dedicated to the lovely ladies in Bay 3, Ward 42, then it was from me. I never heard it as I never listened to hospital radio as I preferred my playlists on my phone, but I trust that it was broadcast.

It was L's birthday during this time. For his birthday, we were supposed to be going canoeing on the River Wye - something he had wanted to do for a long time. There followed a rather factual email on my part explaining why we couldn't go. The company was great and agreed to carry over our booking to such a time as we were all able to go. We still haven't gone - but we will.

H made L a birthday cake which was brought up to the ward that evening. It was delicious and covered in all sorts of goodies - big and small. It was also rather difficult to cut... and little sprinkles went all over my table, bed (!) and the floor. Although the children did their best to pick them up, I imagine the cleaner had more work than she anticipated the next morning. We gave cake to anyone in the bay who wanted some, and their families. The rest was left for all the staff on the night shift. There was none left by the morning so I assume they liked it.

I listened to my music a lot, especially at night when it was difficult to sleep. The beds were pretty comfortable, so that wasn't the problem. We had regular visits from the nurses/HCAs doing their checks. Blood pressure, pulse, temperature and the best one (being on a neuro ward) shining a bright torch in your eyes. This one was pretty hard to sleep through. There was also a particularly loud patient in the men's ward who would come to the nurse's station outside our bay. He would shout and swear very loudly. The nurses were amazing, speaking to him calmly and helping him. Even when he shouted very loud, racist comments to the staff. One male HCA would take him down to the front of the hospital for a cigarette on a regular basis. In the morning, when I asked why they put up with the abuse, the response would always be that the man had a brain injury and didn't know what he was saying. It was not his fault.... Well the respect I had for these amazing people went up even more. The abuse was vitriolic. They would have been absolutely within their rights to say they wouldn't deal with him.

Sleep was a particular problem in the second week. I think it was partly me trying to sort things out in my head and partly the symphony of snores that would be played by the occupants of nearby beds! So I listened to my playlist a lot. Each of the songs has a particular significance to me - either they were ones I like to sing along to, or they were ones we had sung in our choir (so I instantly remembered that particular concert). As my stay in hospital went along, songs were added that sprang to mind in various situations. If you are at all interested in my playlist, it can be found at the end of this story.

Days settled into a routine - mostly based around meals, teas, an injection of clexane (a drug that helped to stop our blood clotting as none of us were moving as much as we would normally (my tummy looked like a dot to dot with all the bruises) and, of course, regular obs. The in-between bits were spent reading, doing puzzles (I completed my first puzzle book from start to finish!), doing jobs that I thought of - usually in the middle of the night when sleep evaded me - and also being an unofficial HCA. I cannot praise the staff at UHCW enough. In the most part, they were fantastic - but also very busy. So I found myself helping the ladies in my bay on many occasions - by pouring water when they couldn't reach their jug, by finding their bell when it got caught down the back of the bed, by shuffling a pillow, opening biscuits.. you name it, I did it. As I have said previously, I felt absolutely fine.

My days were also broken up by lots of lovely visitors. People made the journey from near and far to see me - close friends from home, not so close friends from home, work colleagues, close friends from further away, people who became much closer friends over my time in hospital, I could go on. Many who couldn't visit sent emails or rang. Every bit of contact was appreciated more than you can ever know. You broke up my day and brought cheerfulness and news of the outside world. And on many occasions, you allowed me to escape to the coffee shop or shop downstairs (something I was not allowed to do on my own).

The biggest daily source of joy to me was seeing my family. They came up every evening to see me - after a day at work or a day at school. I have to put in at this point, H had just started her GCSE year and J was 3 days into starting a new school when this happened. To say I worried about the impact this was having on them is putting it mildly. Both schools were told our situation and were very good in terms of the offers of support given. Homework was done in the car on the way up to see me. Poor L would finish work and collect the children from somewhere (home or a friend's house) and then drive up to see me. They often would not get home until nearly 10 after which L would do the admin involved - sending out update emails, confirming who was taking which child to school, who was picking them up and also which visitors were coming that day - and did they need directions? He was - and is - an absolute star.

That is not to say that seeing the family didn't bring its own share of problems. With the power of Google, J had looked up brain tumours and decided that it didn't really matter about looking to the future as I would be dead in 6 months. H, on the other hand, was convinced that during the surgery, they would cut my spinal cord in two and I would be paralysed for the rest of my life. L had to deal with all these thoughts from the children as well as his own fears. I was also reliant on the family to bring me things I asked for. This was incredibly frustrating - I would ask for a certain thing and something else would turn up that they thought would do. It may have done but my frustration at not having what I had asked for is what came through. Unfortunately, most of this frustration would be aimed at, or taken by at any rate, my daughter. Once I was in hospital, she immediately took on the role of housekeeper. She often cooked dinner for L and J. J would then eat it in the car while L ate it on arrival. (If they all didn't use the downstairs Subway). H did all my washing. She would pack the bag that came up to the hospital which contained the random things I had asked for. As I say, my frustrations may or may not have been aimed at her but she took most of them. I apologise profusely for this, H. It was my irritation at the situation that was coming out. I did, and still do, feel guilt at what you had to do then and what you still do now. And I was amazed at how stressful I found discussions about family life. I think this was mainly because I so badly wanted to be at home in the midst of it all.

On the Friday before my op, two things of great significance happened. As you can imagine, having any kind of private conversation between myself and L was all but impossible with the children around. We would send them off to the shop to buy something but this would get us 5 minutes. So on Friday morning, L came to the hospital and the nurses let us go and sit in a small room to talk. We had the "big" talk. We talked about what would happen if I did not make it through the operation. I was always binary about this - I would live or die and not much in-between. We talked about what would happen if I died - I had faith that the children would be Ok as we had such a good support network of friends and family that would look after both him and the children. This was a relief to me. I was not afraid of dying as such at all. I was concerned as to how the last time I would see the children would go. I didn't want their last memory of me to be full of tears. L and I were both adamant that they would both go to school on the Monday. Sitting around at home would do them no good at all. (H was less convinced that this was a good idea!) Writing this now, I have no recollection of talking to L about how he would feel if I died. Guilt is a theme that will run through this story. I feel very guilty now, not to have asked him. We spent a good hour that morning talking about the 'what if's' of Monday and saying our goodbyes (although we would see each other 5 more times before the op!)

That afternoon I was to go for an angiogram. This is a scan that specifically looks at where blood vessels are and would give the surgeons a really good idea of what flowed where, so they could avoid them, if at all possible. I was wheeled down at 4:00pm for this angiogram. A catheter is inserted - this one was in my groin (I don't know if they all are) - and then a series of x-rays are taken. The dye makes the blood vessels show up on an x-ray in a way they wouldn't have without it.

I was told beforehand what would happen. I would be given a local anesthetic and then the catheter would be inserted into my femoral artery. Once this was all OK, the dye would be pumped in and they would take a series of x-rays. Then the catheter would be removed and pressure would be applied to the opening to stop all bleeding. I would be observed for 10 minutes just to make sure all was OK. Occasionally, the wound would start bleeding again, in which case more pressure would be applied for 10 minutes to be sure all bleeding had stopped, after which there would be another 10 minute observation before I was taken up to the ward.

So all went well. Until about 8 minutes into my observations. I suddenly felt warm and wet under my bottom and a nurse said "Quick, her artery's popped". I then spent the next ten minutes with the doctor's elbow pressing very firmly into my groin in order to stop my arterial bleed....

This time was successful and I was eventually returned to the ward. Where I was under close observation and had to lie flat on my back for the first hour, and was gradually allowed to be raised, bit by bit until I could sit upright after four hours (and every 15 minutes, a nurse had to come and look at my groin to check the bleeding hadn't restarted (although with the amount of blood that came out the first time, I think I would have known!) I felt quite embarrassed by nurses (and most frequently a male nurse) continually looking at my groin. I am guessing this examination was to let me in gently - by the time I left hospital, any embarrassment I had of people seeing parts of my body I would rather they didn't, had shrunk considerably.

That night, when I went to the toilet, I was aware of an itchy head and when I looked in the mirror, I thought my face was blotchy but as I didn't have my glasses on, I wasn't too sure.

On Saturday, it was clear I had a rash. It was spreading over my body and I had a very blotchy face. But what was causing it? As a result of the high dose of steroids I was on - in an attempt to shrink the tumour somewhat - my body was unable to control my sugar levels. I had recently been put on insulin. Was it this? Was it something I had eaten? Treatment was obvious - a high, repeated, dose of antihistamines. As to the cause? Who knew? But over the next two days, my body became more and more blotchy. As long as I could still have my operation on Monday, I wasn't too bothered - the rash itself looked pretty spectacular but wasn't too itchy.

On Sunday, I don't remember much. My father came up from Kent to see me over the weekend which was lovely. My mother was ill so was sadly not able to come and visit. I had a variety of other visitors, phone calls and emails. In all of them, I was aware, even if they weren't, that this may be my last communication with them. And of course, on Sunday night I said goodbye to my family. L and I had said our goodbyes to each other on Friday, I wanted the children's last memory of me to be normal, so although we all knew this might be a forever goodbye, to anyone watching, it would have been the same as any other. Though I have to admit to having a long cry once they had gone. And of course my fellow patients knew what had happened and were so supportive once I had had my moments of "privacy".

Monday morning was a beautiful day. I had been nil by mouth since about 4. At 6 I had my usual obs and was sent off to get into my hospital gown. I then spent a couple of hours doing puzzles, emailing L, my parents and a few other people who had emailed me, telling them I was still in the ward and chatting to other patients in the room. One of them was sent off home. One lady, to whom I had spent a lot of time chatting, was taken off for a procedure. I don't think either of us was aware that we wouldn't see each other again. By the time she came back, I would be in theatre; and by the time I came back to the ward in a week or so, she would be at home.

Before my operation I had the customary visit from the anaesthetist. She took one look at my blotchy body and asked what was going on. I told her we didn't know what had caused the allergic reaction but that it wasn't getting any worse. She wrote down another thing to monitor (!) and also said it might make the usual things they wanted to look out for a little more tricky but it should be fine. Phew.

I then had a visit from my consultant, Mr Beltechi. He sat down on my bed and asked me if I had any questions. He held my hand and told me that my operation was not without significant risk to my life.

Did I still want to go ahead? I told him that I didn't think I had much choice - die on an operating table or die when my tumour grew so big that "my sink overflowed" to use their analogy. He agreed with me. I told him that I knew he would do his best for me, and he said he would. Then he said he would see me in theatre.

I was taken down to theatre on my trolley. I went into a room where I saw the anaesthetist again and lots (5?) of other people. I was given an injection into my venflon and told to think of "a happy place". I had expected to be told to count backwards from 10 so this rather threw me. In my mind, I went to somewhere in Cornwall that is beautiful - but would never have expected to be "a happy place". Isn't the mind a weird and wonderful thing?

So my memories of the next few days are rather jumbled. I have large expanses of time about which I remember nothing and then odd memories that apparently are not in the right order.

My first memory is of being back in that favourite place - the tide was in exactly the same state, all was exactly the same. I knew I had had my operation. And had come through? Or was this what it was like on the other side? But I knew I was still alive.

I then remember being in Critical Care. The children were around the bed with my friends B, W and of course L. J asked me if I felt alright. I remember answering "No, half left" - a family joke. I remember counting up to 10 in German. (Can't remember why though) I remember finding it difficult to talk and white gunk coming out of my mouth - which the nurse cleared away for me. I remember her introducing herself and her telling me she would be looking after me and remember thinking/saying she looked just like my boss. Before I had my operation, we took a family picture downstairs which L then printed out. I remember this being stuck to the side of my bed and looking at that. I remember taking my oxygen off because it made my mouth dry and being told to put it on again as my SATS were dropping. And I remember having a dry, dry mouth. Oh boy do I remember that. I was given a top tip - to get a wet piece of gauze and to wipe my lips/mouth with it. It brought temporary relief and would for weeks to come. Swabs were my best friend!

And I remember waking one night as a fellow patient in the room's heart stopped. The staff came round to use the defibrillator to resuscitate him. This was successful. Until his heart stopped again a short while later - and he was resuscitated again. He was then moved into theatre. I obviously never knew what happened to him. I remember thinking that this was far calmer than it was portrayed in Casualty!

I was then moved to Step Down. This was a room on the Neurological Ward which was part way between Critical Care and the normal bay. This meant that there was one nurse for four of us rather than one nurse for six of us in the normal bay and one to one nurse to patient care in Critical Care. During this time, I was only allowed to be flat on my back to allow the wound in my skull to have some time to get used to the hole left by my tumour debulking. (As there was a very small bit of tumour left in there (which I had been told would be likely, due to the tricky position of the tumour), it was called a debulking of the tumour rather than a removal (when all of the tumour is taken out)). It was becoming apparent that I could not talk very well. Was this down to the anaesthetic tubing or something else? I was being tube fed. I still had a catheter in and was wearing pads. (This is the grown up word for nappies…..) I was being given lactulose. This loosens the bowels as I was not able to move around and there was a danger I would become constipated. Well, I shall leave you to put two and two together. It was not pleasant. I think it was in Step Down that I devised the term Shitty Saturday. Things always seemed to be worse on Saturdays - for quite a few weeks to come. Saturdays seemed to be a day which was physically and mentally tough. I remember two of my closest friends coming to visit me on that first Saturday. All I can say is that it is a good job they have known me for many, many years. I think I was very grumpy that day - wanting to sit up mostly as I was fed up of lying on my back. The ceiling tiles within my sight were not very interesting!! But I counted them frequently...

One of my other memories of being in Step Down was having my sheets changed. This was something that was done every day and was lovely. But I remember being asked to lift my head and not being able to. It felt like it weighed about 15 stone. The HCA's were rather less careful about lifting it up and putting it down than they might have been...

And a story that still makes me smile! One day, I was having a particularly bad morning - lots of moaning and tears. L was on the receiving end of this and decided to come and see me. Although visiting hours were quite strict - a couple of hours in the afternoon and a couple of hours in the evening - partners were allowed to come in the mornings too as long as they weren't in the bays for meal times. So L turned up at the hospital. And there was a great spreading of rumours. "The CQC are here and coming up to ward 42." There was great relief when it was only Mr T coming to see Lucinda. His lanyard from work was the same colour as that from the CQC who often did unannounced inspections!!

On 1st October, I was helped to sit up in a chair. This was a very slow procedure. I had been slowly allowed to sit up in bed the day before so the health care staff were happy that nothing dreadful would happen within my skull. It was great to be able to sit in my hospital chair - something normal that I used to be able to do. But oh my goodness…. half an hour of sitting out of bed and I was totally exhausted!!!

Shortly after this, I was deemed well enough to move into the bay in which I had started in. Wow! This felt like such an achievement..

I must have spent about five weeks in this bay before moving on again.

Over several days, my dressings were reduced and eventually, my staples taken out. However, after a few days, my wound was itchy and H said it looked a bit grim. Nurses were called to look at it. I would have gunk on my pillow regularly. After a few days, the consultants were concerned enough to take some action. My wound was infected. The first attempt to sort it out was to get the plastic surgeon nurse involved. She came and slathered it in manuka honey strips. This made my wound, my hair and my pillow very sticky. It was also at about this time that I started having very intense pains down the left side of my face. At this stage, they would occur every 60 seconds or so and this would go on for several hours. The consultants decided that they would need to clean out my wound in theatre. I was sent for a scan to see whether the infection had gone into my skull - this would require another craniotomy (removal of part of the skull). The scan showed that the infection was just superficial so would just need debriding (given a good clean out with dead skin either side of the wound removed) and stapling back together. This would also require a plastic surgeon in theatre as the wound was so long....

Day by day, I grew stronger, slowly but surely. I would get regular physio and eventually, I was able to get myself out of bed and into my chair and back again with only the help of a piece of equipment called an ETAC. And doing this brings me to one of my worst moments in hospital. I had called for assistance to help me get from the bed to the chair and after a while called for some help to get back again (if nothing else, I needed the equipment to help me.) I rang my bell, and asked for some help. The nurse who came to help me said "Why can't you do it yourself? I'm not paid enough to do manual labour." I burst into tears and said "I would if I could but I can't". At this point the doctors popped their heads around the curtains - they were doing their daily round. I was asked if I was OK to which I responded "No". The doctor said she would see how I was doing tomorrow and if I wanted any psychological help. The team of Doctors heard the nurses response to me. I don't know what happened after that but I know that, thankfully, that nurse was never on duty in my bay for the rest of my time there. As I say, this was a rare occurrence of care that was not great.

During this time, when movement was limited - and for many weeks after - my life could be found inside a Tesco value tissue box! In it would be my phone, headphones, lip balm, wet gauze and of course tissues. I would have this within my reach, day and night and woe betide anyone who moved it away from me when changing my sheets or washing me!

There were some very interesting people in the bay with me. Two of them were long term residents like myself. Over the weeks, we formed a great relationship and relied on each other for support many times. We had some more interesting residents. All of whom, I hasten to add, had brain injuries. Although my recovery has been long, and difficult at times, I thank my lucky stars that I came out of surgery with all my mental faculties (mostly) intact. The lady on my right side for a week or so was deaf in her left ear. As I still had very little volume in my voice, she would talk to me, I would answer and she wouldn't hear. She was a very unhappy patient for a number of reasons but I would get very upset when she had visitors and she would be crying to them and telling them that she was so disliked in the bay that even her neighbour wouldn't talk to her!!

Another resident in the bay was again very unhappy. She would express her anger at being there by throwing things. Including an (empty) cup, then a (full) cup of tea, a nearly empty jug and finally a full jug. All at my visitors or me. I don't think this was intentional but let's just say that her aim was improving, the longer she stayed in the bay. And as she often removed a soiled pad when it became uncomfortable, I was becoming more than slightly nervous....She was then moved to a private room so she could throw to her heart's content. This is a top tip for you - if you want to be moved to a private room, cause problems for the other residents in your bay! Well this was certainly the case when I was there.

The investigations into why I couldn't talk well carried on. Each week SALT (Speech and Language Team) would come to see me. They are in fact the people who have the most power over the most important thing to me (and to fellow patients) - eating! They were the people that would tell me when I could eat food again. Because as well as not being able to speak very well, I was still being fed by my NG (NasoGastric tube). Each week, I would have a camera passed through my nose and down to the back of my throat to see what was going on. This also involved drinking blue milk and a variety of foods with increasingly thick consistencies. The first time this happened, it was established that my left vocal cord was paralysed. This was the explanation for why I couldn't talk well. But was this caused by a bleed (there was nothing in my notes to suggest this) or as a result of the anaesthetic and associated tubing causing inflammation? I was given lots of physio exercises for my vocal cords and neck and told the SALT team would be back next week. Their visits were eagerly anticipated - I was desperate to be able to get rid of the NG tube and eat normal meals. Each week I was disappointed - it was still not safe for me to swallow so I needed to have my nutrition via the bag. The main concern was that I would pass food or drink into my lungs rather than my stomach and I could then come down with a lung infection.

Being fed by a tube had all sorts of problems associated with it. I didn't find it uncomfortable which was good. But it did mean that I couldn't go very far. At the start, I would have my "food" in a couple of meals. When I was bed bound, this didn't cause me any issues. All my drugs needed to be pulverised and then water was added so that they could be sent up my tube. But there was one problem. Only nurses who had "got the certificate" were able to give me my drugs through the tube or even give me my food. During the week, this was not a problem. But at the weekends, this was more of an issue. There were fewer staff on duty, and often the member of staff that was in charge of our bay was a locum member of staff who did not have the ticket and although they had done the work involved in NG tube administration, were not insured by the trust to do this. So we had to wait for an insured nurse to come. On one weekend, it must have been very busy. My drugs had been put out of my reach (and also out of sight). My food was connected up, but late. I was starving! But my drugs weren't administered. The next day, I had an apology from one of the nurses. They had found my drugs and realised that I hadn't been given any pain relief for 24 hours. That would explain why I had been feeling so rotten!

The other problem with being tube fed was what happened if the tube came out. It obviously needed to be reinserted. This was not particularly pleasant but not something I found painful. If it was reinserted, then several tests needed to happen. It needed to go into the stomach rather than the lungs so the tube needed to go in a certain length.

Before every feed was connected, and if the tube had come out and was re-inserted, the nurse needed to check my aspirate. This involved syringing out some of my stomach contents. If the pH was less than 5, then the tube was obviously in my stomach and we were good to go. If it was 5.5 or above..... then they could test the aspirate twice more. If it was 7 or above, I would need to have an xray to check the tube was in the correct place. So aspirate testing became a tense moment. Particularly if I had had the tube reinserted. Sometimes no aspirate could be syringed out. And then all sorts of games were played. Lie on a different side to move the stomach contents around. Jiggle around to make sure your stomach juices were all around your stomach. Have a drink (when I was allowed to) to dilute the stomach juices (but also the pH...). It was a tense time of the day. So if my aspirate was not of the required pH, I needed to go and have an x-ray to check it was in the right place. And as my food was very often set up in the evening, I would be sent to the radiology department in the evening. And there was often a queue. So on at least three occasions, I had to wait until after midnight to go down to have the x-ray. Then it needed to be looked at by a Doctor (and there were not many of those around on the night shift). And if it was all ok, I would finally get my food between 1 and 2 in the morning. (And my night time drugs...) By this time I would be both starving and in pain.

When you are in hospital, particularly when you are bed bound, you are at the complete mercy of the staff. As I have said, for the most part they were fantastic. There was one night shift HCA who had clear favourites. If you were one of her favourites, then all was fine. But if you weren't.... Fairly soon into my stay on Ward 42 (although at the time it seemed like ages after the operation), it was my son's 12th birthday. Fairly soon after the operation, I had said to him that I was sure that I would be that I would be home by then to celebrate his birthday. As it happened, I still couldn't walk, talk properly or eat so this wasn't going to happen. However, my husband arranged for him and the children to stay the night in a local hotel. It is the tradition in our house that we all gather on mine and my husband's bed to open presents at the start of the day. So we talked to the staff and they said we could have a room and they would help to get me ready to go and watch him open his presents before school. This all happened and the HCA mentioned above was the one who came to help me get dressed and into the wheelchair. She was lovely - so kind and helpful. A few nights later, an incident occured. When the day staff came in, I had not been washed or changed and my "pad" was very full - leaking even. The day staff were appalled. The night staff were spoken to when they came on shift. I was asked why I hadn't asked for a bedpan (the reason being I had slept through the night for the first time). From that moment on, the HCA treated me dreadfully. She would come and give me a bedpan and clean me without uttering a word. She was rude - not only to me but to other people in the bay whom she deemed had upset her. We came to dread the nights when she was on duty. Thankfully, I moved to the next door ward shortly after this incident so didn't see her for much longer. But on the other hand, one day a different HCA accidentally pulled out my NGA tube. She was so apologetic and treated me so well every shift afterwards.

I was still having regular MRI scans at this point and so got to know some of the porters pretty well too. They were also lovely and always tried to cheer us patients up. On my way to a scan, one of them said "Oh, do you know your pyjamas are covered in poo?" I looked down with complete alarm and the two porters had a good chuckle. I had been bought some lovely WInnie the Pooh pyjamas. And the bottoms were covered in lots of Pooh bears....! I did find it funny once the original shock had worn off!

During my time in this ward, I was slowly getting stronger. I was able to get myself out of bed and into my chair. And back again. I had had my catheter removed. This brought it's own issues. I now needed to get myself to the toilet on time. I was able to walk to the toilet first with two nurses, then with one, and then, excitement of excitements, I was given my very own zimmer frame to use. Oh, the feelings of joy. And independence. Going with nurses was great - but you needed to ring your bell in enough time for them to come and help you and you to get to the toilet. At night, when I was connected to the NG tube and there were fewer staff around, I still had to use the bedpan. And again, you needed to ring the bell and speak to someone well in advance of actually having to go to the loo. With my zimmer frame, I could now walk to the window or walk to the beds of my friends to have a chat and get some exercise - or go to the toilet!

My rash had gone. After many investigations, it was thought to be a reaction to the contrast dye used in my angiogram. A lot of people had allergic reactions to it - although not on that scale! I definitely had left-sided weakness but a bigger problem for me was the lack of proprioception in my left side. Proprioception is the brain's awareness of where parts of the body are. In my case, my brain was struggling to place my hand and foot. I spent many hours whilst in bed trying to firstly touch and secondly pick up my cup. And when it came to walking, trying to put my foot in the right place! This was exhausting. On many occasions, I felt like a toddler. And now I realise why they need so much sleep! (As long as no one asked me to crawl, I'd be alright....) Another odd thing about post-op me was that I had no feelings of pain or temperature on the right side of my body.... Useful for when blood was taken but everyone said it was a little peculiar! And I had a name for the other things that weren't right. Ataxia. A condition that may affect balance and walking, speaking, swallowing, tasks that require a great deal of control such as writing and eating and vision. Well, I could write and my vision was ok but otherwise, everything fit. And I now have a very wonky tongue! The cause? A brain tumour or a stroke. A tick to both of those. The cure? There isn't one but symptoms should improve with physiotherapy.

Talk was now being made of moving me. Either to the Rehab ward next door or to The Alexandra Hospital. If I was moved to The Alex, it would be far easier for friends and family to visit. But we were waiting for a bed. Or I could go next door and get specialised Neuro Rehab physio, but it was still quite a trek for friends and family to visit. But we were waiting for a bed. My preference was to stay at UHCW as the ward next door specialised in Neuro rehab. But if a bed came up at The Alex, then who knew what decision would be made? Enough progress had been made that there was no longer talk of sending me to a specialised rehab hospital in town halfway between home and UHCW.

My family came to visit me pretty much every day. They did my washing, brought me things I needed, helped wheel me downstairs in the wheelchair, and cheered my spirits no end. There were many occasions where they would arrive and one or other of them would disappear downstairs to get their dinner from Subway! My son found it difficult to see me in this state I think. He would come and say hello, talk for a few minutes and then go to the relative's room to watch telly. This was his way of coping with a pretty unusual and difficult situation. When I look back at the photos of me, I cannot blame him. I looked horrendous (so much so that one friend told me, when I was out of hospital, that I was looking so much better. And every time she had come to see me when I was in hospital, she had thought I was going to die!!!) We tried to explain to the children that we didn't know how much better I would get. Perhaps I would make a complete recovery, but most likely I wouldn't. But there may be some things about me that would be better than pre-op. It was a bit like doing a computer reboot.

H was always very attentive to me. She would like to be a nurse when she has finished school and if my care was anything to go by, she will make a fantastic one. She would take off my compression socks, massage my feet with a nice lotion, before putting them back on again; she would help me to the toilet if needed, and she would regularly comb and style (?) what was left of my hair. Lots of it was falling out every day and there was obviously a large area that had been shaved for the operation. It was while doing this one evening that she found a random staple in my head. All of the staples around my wound had long been removed, and this was half way up my head - on the opposite side!! The bell was rung and a nurse removed the staple. She was rather confused too! As well as hair coming out, I was also losing lots of skin. When I spoke to the Doctor, she put me on vitamin B supplements. It is not usual for someone to spend so long being tube fed and the feed didn't have all the required vitamins I guess. The feeds have a good balance of protein, carbohydrates and fibre. Amounts were adjusted each week depending on what I was doing, how much I weighed and what number I gave when I opened my bowels! After a few days, my hair and skin stopped getting worse but it was several months before they started getting better.

Two significant occasions happened while I was in Ward 42. The first was my son's 12th birthday. We celebrated the start of this with present opening together. This was lovely - but did mean that I slept for most of the day! My daughter made an amazing cake for him and a few friends. And she arranged the trip to a trampoline park and then the sleep over - with some support from L and my mother-in-law. I missed being involved with something that I would usually organise.

The second was one that didn't really enter my radar until about 10 days before hand. Half term... Now as I work in education, this was something that we had never really had to think about...I would be around to entertain/supervise/referee/chauffeur... and while I was happy to leave the children on their own for a few hours in the evening, all day for five days was a bit much. L's work were being great about allowing him to work flexible hours when needed but we didn't want to use up holiday if we didn't need to (who knew what we might need in the next few weeks?) or use up more goodwill. Both sets of grandparents had been great over the last month staying at the house, sending food parcels and offering emotional support and now they both came to the rescue with childcare over half term. Thank you, thank you thank you.

My mental state was also made a lot better by the on-going and frequent visits of friends - I generally had two a day. I would have a visitor (or sometimes even two) at afternoon visiting times and then often a visitor at the start of evening visiting before the family arrived. To all of you who came to visit -sometimes also collecting the children from random places and bringing them with you too, sent emails, rang, sent letters, sent cards and/or presents, you made my life in hospital so much more pleasant. And to those of you who couldn't manage to visit but helped out with taking the children to school, collecting them, looking after J when he couldn't face coming up to the hospital again, cooking for the family and so many other things, I thank you from the bottom of my heart.

Another thing that still puts a smile on my face was a recording sent to me from the conductor of the choir I sing in (notorious). When they heard of my news (L sings in the choir too so passed on what was happening when he felt able to), they all gathered round the piano for an impromptu singing of the theme tune to Friends (a piece we had done a couple of years earlier) - no music for anyone - and recorded it for me. Whenever I hear it, I always grin. Thank you.

L was, and still is, a rock. He was having to deal with my emotions - a lot of frustration, but also tiredness and general grumpiness - and also with the children's. They did not miss a day of school throughout this whole story. This is due to their commitment to school but also due to L talking patiently through all their questions and issues. A lot of these questions would be asked in the car on the way home - so at about 9pm. Everyone was tired. I just had to go to sleep after they had gone. L still had a whole lot of work to do. And when they got home, he would check the pick-ups and drop-offs for the children and certainly, in the early days. reply to emails asking how I was. When he tells me of some of the conversations he had with the children, or some of the potential ones (How do I tell the children their mother has died?), I think I may have had the easier job, I knew I just had to keep on doing my physio and slowly but surely making progress. He had all the mental side of things to cope with. When I looked at my fellow patients who had lost mental capacity following a brain injury, I thank my lucky stars I lost physical capacity. It would have been so much harder to have to try to regain my brain than to make progress using my body. Although I am still not back to my pre-op physical self, I can adapt to that life. But I can still read, write, go to work and remember things with the family - so important.

Eventually, there was a space in the next door ward - Ward 43, Neurological Rehabilitation. This meant a lot more physio, so hopefully a speedier recovery and quicker home time. I had already told J that I would be home for his birthday and missed that one by quite a bit. We were also planning a couple of nights away with some friends and their families. This was to be at half term. I was hopeful that I would be able to come out for the day at least. But no. I missed that one too. So now, I was hoping to be home for Christmas. But didn't want to say too much to the children in case that deadline came and went too.

But with more physio came quicker progress. While November was the month of the zimmer frame.,December was the month of crutches - another huge milestone. For any distance longer than my bed to the end of the ward, I needed the use of a wheelchair. But within the ward, I could use two crutches. What freedom! And they are a lot easier to work around when in the bathroom too! Each day I was taken - or walked - up to the gym. Here I had exercises to improve my strength but mostly my proprioception. I was given equipment to do my exercises with on my bed.

When I arrived in Ward 43, I was still being NG fed. I was now allowed one long feed overnight. But I still encountered the same problems with regard to nurses who were "ticketed" to hook it all up. I needed a long feed - and the nursing changeover was during visiting hours. So did I get connected in the day shift? Quick and easy - but then I couldn't leave the ward with the family. Or did I wait til I got back from my trip out and hope that the nurse assigned to our bay was insured by the trust to connect me up? I would make my decisions based on how tired I was on any particular day.

Although I still wasn't allowed to eat anything, the SALT team had decided that I was sensible enough to be able to have sips of water. After a while, I was able to take several sips at a time and had progressed to apple and mango squash, (yum) dissolved marmite in hot water (wow) and tea (a bit of an anticlimax as it was never made with boiling water). One Saturday, a nurse came on duty and took pity on me. She said that if I was able to drink all these drinks, I should be able to drink soup. That day, things changed for me. I had a cup of thin, chicken soup for my lunch. Heaven. The next day, it was thin mushroom soup. Wow! On Monday, the nurse on duty was informed of what had happened regarding my lunches and was not prepared to sanction this unless SALT had been consulted. SALT duly arrived, and the camera was stuck up my nose again. They were still not 100% happy but as I had already been having some soup and if I promised them I would go slowly, they would progress me to a puree diet. I never thought I would be so pleased to eat purees!! Again, it was like being a baby/toddler! I soon worked out that pureed meat was pretty grim!! (One of the worst meals was roast chicken!) Pureed fish was ok and vegetables were good. I was very amused to find that the food would come moulded to look like what it was supposed to be - peas pureed and then moulded to look like peas. I would take a picture of my food each day and post on facebook so friends could guess what I was having. For my last 10 days in hospital, I was promoted to a "fork-mashable" diet. Before going on this, I had to sign a disclaimer saying that I knew it was against their advice. The team were still not totally happy that I wouldn't choke on the small bits in my food. Once again, I promised to go slowly and they agreed to let me give it a go.

And the day before I left, I was allowed to eat a normal diet! (But as we had to order our food 24 hours in advance, I didn't get to enjoy this)

As always, I had fellow room-mates. The lady to the left of me when I arrived was a lovely lady. I want to say she suffered from dementia. But while she certainly had dementia, I can't say she was suffering. She was one of the happiest people I have ever met. Every morning she would wake up and open her curtains. She would then name every bird she saw and would talk to them all day. She told me all about her boyfriend who would come to visit her every day to check she was OK. Her only concern was that he wouldn't know she was in hospital. He was actually a health care worker. She was waiting for a room in the next door dementia unit in which she was a regular visitor. Then she would be deemed well enough to go back to her flat. After which she would be admitted back to the Neuro ward for a variety of reasons (usually to do with not drinking enough) before the cycle would begin again. She also spent her day singing. Her repertoire was limited - but was made up of songs my grandmother used to sing so I would find it very comforting.

She was then followed by another lovely lady. This lady was a Doctor - as she kept telling all the medics who came to look after. And there is nothing like saying you are a Doctor to make sure that the consultants see you quickly and you are given excellent treatment. That is not to say I wasn't given excellent treatment, but her bed was always changed first and she was always given first choice of yogurt and things. It was only after quite a few days that I realised she was not a medical doctor but an academic one. And it was a few more days before the staff realised this!

There was another lady in our bay who was slightly scarier. She was in our bay because she had had a fall and they wanted to check there was nothing sinister going on. She was an alcoholic and had come to hospital with a very high blood alcohol level - almost certainly the cause of her fall. And was now having severe withdrawal symptoms, which led to some pretty angry outbursts. At other times, she was sweet as sweet could be. She was also a smoker. Her cigarettes and a lighter were confiscated fairly quickly (but given back to her when she went out for a smoke). However she had a second lighter that the staff didn't know about. I remember a rather alarming evening when she threatened to use her lighter. And as the lady in the next bed was on oxygen, this could have had rather dramatic results! This lighter was then also confiscated by the nursing staff. I also remember one night when I went to the toilet. I came back to find her in my bed and looking through all my belongings for the lighter I had stolen! After several minutes, the night staff managed to send her back to her bed. But I was rather more wary of going to the loo in the night after that experience.

The ward I was in was a Neuro Rehab ward. This meant that we were all being geared up to going home. But to do this, there were several people who needed to be satisfied that I was ready to cope on my own. In due course, a meeting would be had with several interested parties and a potential discharge date would be set.

My days were filled with visits from physios and/or doing my exercises. Physio involved practicing walking with my zimmer at first and then crutches. Or being wheeled to the physio room and practising walking up a step or being given exercises to strengthen my legs. As the days progressed and there was talk of me going home, we moved to the stairwell and tried various methods for tackling the stairs. This required a lot of concentration as much as anything else..!!

I then had a couple of visits from the Neuro Psychology team. The first member turned up at 7:30 one morning asking if he could chat to me for half an hour or so. I hadn't even been to the loo! I told him I was happy to talk to him once I had had a wee and as long as he was aware that I had just woken up! We had a great chat. He asked me to do lots of puzzles which I loved - and think I did well at. There are quite a few that I will do with the children I work with when there is a spare few minutes and some that make great car games. He then asked if he could send a colleague to do a few more activities that were a bit trickier. This was the most fun I had had in weeks - absolutely yes. She came at lunchtime so I was actually awake! I am proud to say that I did her activity quicker than anyone she had seen.

(It did help that I had posed a similar question to some students when I used to teach science. I told her this and she said it was fine and showed that that bit of my brain was still working well.)

I also had regular visits from the occupational therapist who wanted to check that I would be able to manage once I returned home. This involved a long page of measurements that L had to make of our home. This was then cross-referenced with the physios who checked I would be able to climb a stair of x cm. We made a few adaptations to our home. Firstly, there was a question about whether I would be able to climb the step at the front of the house and actually get in. My father-in-law then built a ramp out of plywood that meant I could get into and over the step at the front of the house. Tick. We have a downstairs toilet so that was OK - and a seat was ordered from a County mobility hire scheme that raised it a bit so I didn't have to lean on the basin in order to stand up. L managed to get hold of a bed so I could sleep in the study downstairs. So that was set up - as well as moving the computer and desk upstairs! Tick. I was able to climb stairs with the help of a rail - which we didn't have. So L fixed one of those. Tick. And as I couldn't walk without a stick, a kitchen trolley was borrowed from the mobility hire scheme so I could make myself a drink or some lunch and get it from the kitchen to the sitting room. Tick. And she needed to see if I could take care of my personal hygiene. So there followed a visit to the toilet (fully clothed) to check I could sit, stand and put my hands in the appropriate places. Yup. Could I clean my teeth and brush my hair? Yes, she could watch me doing those. Could I wash myself? So it was arranged that she would come and watch me having a shower and washing my hair. Well, I can't say I felt at all comfortable having someone watch me shower and wash, but I did it. She did say afterwards that she had never seen anyone have a shower quite so quickly! And then I said that I bathed more than showered at home. Why oh why? Thankfully the getting in and out of the bath practice was done fully clothed. As far as she was concerned, I was now ready to go home.

I had several trips out of hospital over the last few weeks. My first was a day out, locally. So the family came up, we packed up my stuff (wheelchair, warm clothes, my handbag (what was that and what was it used for?) and we set off after breakfast to the local B&M and did some Christmas shopping...! This was followed by a visit to IKEA - mainly to get a mattress for my bed. We had lunch here. I tried some sweet potato fries - they are nice and soft aren't they? Well it turns out fries were something that I struggled to eat that day and for many months to come! After a quick visit to local TKMaxx for some more Christmas shopping, I was returned to the hospital - absolutely exhausted but very happy to have had a mostly successful trip out of the hospital. I had negotiated getting in and out of the car, shopping and going to the toilet in a strange place amongst other things. Wow! What a feeling of achievement. And wonderful to be doing normal things with the family.

My next trip out was a day visit home. This was partly to check how things would work out at home. Oh my goodness, I had forgotten what it was like to go hurtling down a dual carriageway at what felt like 100mph tailgating every other car on the road...It was pretty scary!! Our friends, B and M, popped round. And I proudly made them cups of tea and coffee. (I couldn't carry them through from the kitchen, but I did make them). I managed to eat some soup for lunch, and again have some normal family time.

The next hurdle was the Team Meeting. I was desperate to go home now. I had had a taste of freedom and great though the hospital staff were, I wanted to go home. Primarily so I could be a Mum to my children again (this was difficult in hospital - H spent a lot of her time looking after me (which I knew would continue at home too but hopefully in a different way) and J was finding it ever harder to see me (he wanted answers about when I would come home - answers we just couldn't give him). So the meeting was arranged.

There would be me, and L, my consultant, someone from physio, from OT and someone from the neuro psychology department. Firstly, the psychologist said I was of sound mind and able to contribute to the discussion and my opinions were valid and made by someone capable of making the decision. OT said she was happy for me to go home - with the adaptations that had been discussed. Physio said that they had a list of criteria I had to fulfill before going. The consultant said he would like me to go just after Christmas. I said I was going before then. He said maybe a couple of days before. I wanted to go the next week (the last weekend of November). This was not received well! I said I wanted a few days at home before the children broke up from school so I could get used to things. This caused a few more raised eyebrows... We agreed on the second week of December - providing physio were happy that I had completed their checklist, coped with a weekend at home and nothing untoward happened either in hospital or at home.

I can tell you that nothing was going to stop me ticking off their checklist!

The weekend at home went well. If I was exhausted, so what? I was exhausted at home.

And so on Friday December 7th, the day before my 45th birthday, I finally went home. For good!

Life at home was good - but tiring. The weekend was spent trying to work out what I could do on my own at home and what I might need to leave. I soon realised I needed a set of boxes filled with things I might need or want such as tissues, books, puzzle books, snacks (that were soft - I still couldn't eat reliably well) and phone chargers - pretty much an expanded tissue box.

On Monday, I was left on my own. Yikes. I settled in on the sofa. It had been arranged that various friends would pop in to say hello and see if I needed anything. This worked well. And of course I still needed a good long sleep during the day. The children were being taken to school by the same families that took them while I was in hospital. So that routine was able to carry on. H was very concerned as to my well-being and would text several times a day to check I was OK.

One night, early on, J came to see me in my bed downstairs. He snuggled up for a cuddle and then shed a tear about a problem he was having at school. THIS was why I wanted to be at home. To be able to be a Mum to H and J. It might be trickier to get around at home than at hospital, but this was where I wanted to be. And I would get better here, just in a different way and at a different pace.

On my birthday, it was the Notorious concert. This was definitely something I wanted to attend. L was singing in it and it was something normal to do. But as L had a rehearsal in the afternoon and I couldn't drive, the only realistic option was for me and the children to go into Birmingham for the afternoon while L rehearsed. So a trip was planned to The Sealife Centre. J has always had a thing for marine biology so this seemed apt. We turned up at the centre. One good thing about being in a wheelchair, H got in as a carer and I got in free. Bargain - even if she did have to push me round! Afterwards, we went to Costa for a hot chocolate. This was a first for me... And then we loitered with intent waiting for L to come and pick us up. Finally we were collected and went off to the church. This was not possible to go into in a wheelchair - and I didn't want to use it anyway. So I waddled in using my crutches and we set up base at the back of the church. It was so lovely to see all my singing friends. And I even had a song dedicated to me - I'll be Home for Christmas. That really made my evening, and birthday. But boy was I tired!!

Over the next couple of weeks, we did lots of the usual Christmas things - bought and decorated the tree, put up the Christmas cards, planned our Christmas dinner. This was a nice change. Usually, we visit one set or other of parents for Christmas. This year, we were staying at home. So different, but good. H had to do most of the cooking, with a bit of help from L. I cautiously ate my share of dinner, and it was excellent.

There was one significant change to our usual, pre-Christmas routine. We usually have all our neighbours round for drinks on the Saturday before Christmas. This year, some other neighbours volunteered to host which was a relief in the end (although I had harboured a desire to still host this for quite a few weeks! In the end, head gave way to heart and I agreed to let them host). I made it up the road to see everybody. And while most of the neighbours had caught up on the happenings in our house over the last few months, there were still a few who were unaware.

Being at home with the family was great, after all these weeks. But was not without difficulties for me. Having been the lynch-pin of the family for so long, they had all got on without me for 12 weeks. And things were being done differently and I found I didn't really like it. There were new routines, different people were doing things, and it was all OK. But hard for me. I had always been the person who organised meals, sorted out packed lunches, did the shopping and generally knew what was happening and when in our house. And now different people were doing them and doing them well. Where was my place in the family?

PART 2

2019 - Year of Recovery

So, I was home. What next?

Over the year, I made slow but steady progress. There are many people who helped with this, but overall the progress I made was down to my will and determination to get better. As mentioned previously, ataxia is incurable. But improvements can be made with physio and hard work and now, looking back, I am so much better than I was in January 2019.

On leaving hospital, I knew I had been referred to the Worcestershire Acute Trust for: speech therapy, occupational health and physio and for my rehabilitation consultant. All of these would be easier for me to access as several would be at my local hospital. So the waiting began. I was told that the waiting list for neuro physio was about 12 weeks. The same amount of time that I had been in hospital. But my theory was that if I was doing things around the house, then that was physio of sorts too - and getting me to where I wanted to be. I also started back at choir - although singing alto not soprano and with a limited range, and started back at governance. Both of these improved my mental health immeasurably as I was back to doing something normal.

The one set of appointments that were still, and always will be, at UHCW are my check-ups on my brain tumour. One of the disadvantages of meningiomas is that they are likely to grow back again. And as mine has been debulked rather than removed, I suppose this is even more likely. However, they are very slow growing. As such, no one could tell me how long mine had been there for. 5 years? 10 years? 25 years?

So, I return to UHCW for my checkups. These are every six months to start off with and will reduce to every year after a while. These appointments are preceded by an MRI scan to check the growth of the tumour.

My first checkup was six weeks after discharge. It was with Mr Beltechi and was very informative. And quite scary. It was mine and L's first time to ask questions, with my having made a successful recovery. We were shown scans of the tumour site then and now. What amazed me was how much my spinal cord had been pushed out of the way by the tumour. What struck L the most was the way he kept shaking his head and saying how difficult it had all been. He was amazed that I was walking, talking and eating again. This meant the operation was a big success. The tumour had completely surrounded 1 of the 4 arteries that give the brain blood and 2 of the veins that take blood away from the brain. And all the nerves to do the eating, drinking, swallowing, vision and breathing among other things. He also explained that the hole that had been made in my skull to get rid of the tumour was about 7cm by 7cm (so about 50cm^2). This was covered in a mesh and over time, my skull would grow back over this. So, if I fall over, best not fall over onto that part of my head....!

I told him about the shooting pains I was still getting - on a daily basis - in my head. He said that the likely cause was nerve irritation. This may or may not go away. He recommended a couple of painkillers.

As to the next step if the tumour came back? This would be radiotherapy rather than surgery. I would be scanned regularly enough that if it did start growing back, it would be caught early enough for this to be the best option. The radiotherapy itself would cause some nerve damage so he wanted to leave this until it was absolutely needed so that I could recover as much as possible before starting this treatment. At least it seemed highly unlikely that I would need to have brain surgery again. Phew

One evening at choir, a fellow singer, who worked with the speech therapy department at Worcester Royal Hospital said she had seen my referral to speech therapy and was going to be managing my treatment if that was OK. Soon I was asked to go to WRH where I had another scan on my vocal cords. The left one was still paralysed. But there was a possible solution that would help matters if I wanted to give it a go….. Botox. Apparently this made the vocal cord bigger, thus enabling them to meet - and my voice to get better. This would not be a permanent solution but would certainly give me more volume in the short term and may improve my range. This could be repeated up to twice more if needed/ wanted and after that it was surgery. Surgery is not something that appealed to me then, and still doesn't. My hope was that gradually I would be able to exercise the vocal cord enough for there to be no need for another injection. I was also referred for speech therapy. This took place over several weeks at The Alex. It turns out that lots of the exercises I was given are very similar to those we do at choir. Bonus.. As to the botox; there was an instant improvement in my voice - as soon as I picked up the children from friends, they noticed it. When I spoke on the phone it was much clearer. (Indeed, one friend said he would now start phoning me again - he had stopped doing this in the last few months as he was worried that I would answer the phone and he wouldn't be able to hear me!) So straight away, one aspect of my recovery was measurable.

There are two other health professionals who have aided my recovery. Lisa is someone I knew pre-op as H had been to her for some physio and also some work experience. I have been to see her every month. She gives my back, neck and shoulders a massage and helps to loosen off my (very tight) muscles. This provides enormous relief and gives me much greater movement. We also have a good chat and laugh about things so is good for my mental health too.

Which brings me onto Di. Di had the unenviable task of trying to help me sort out what was going on inside my head. At one of my appointments with my GP, it was suggested that I might benefit from talking to a professional about the events of the previous six months. Di helped me work through many feelings and also suggested that I write my story. So you can thank her for this!

If I was going out with the family, I was using a wheelchair. Although I could get around the house with a stick or two, and I could get to the car, anything further than that was very tiring. Being in a wheelchair had advantages - I could go out with the family, people would tend not to crash into me in the way that they did if I was walking with my sticks - and of course there were handles from which to hang bags.

But it also came with disadvantages. As I am sure any user of a wheelchair can agree with, being in a wheelchair renders you invisible to many people. Conversations between family members would be had over my head and I couldn't hear them. If we met somebody in the shops, they would talk to whoever was pushing me rather than me. When we were in a shop, I was dependent on whoever was pushing me to stop where I wanted to stop - and not having much voice at this stage meant they couldn't hear me..... (and the brain surgery didn't leave me with the ability to send messages telepathically) So I was very keen to stop using it as soon as possible.

Luckily, we have private health insurance through my husband's work. So the search began for a neuro physiotherapist. It turns out there aren't too many in the Birmingham area. Add to that, the fact that I couldn't drive. The search was frustrating to say the least. And when we did find one that seemed to fit our criteria (a physio who worked with neuro patients and wasn't too far away) I would ring them to find out they had moved to New Zealand or had retired. It seemed that I would have to hold on until the NHS system kicked in to place. As many people said to me: The NHS is great in a crisis but not so great for chronic conditions.

Then one day L came home saying he had found a neuro physio who not only was local but would come to the house. This sounded too good to be true. So L rang her and checked that what he had found out was true. She was not listed as someone that the insurers would cover, but they thought they could sort this out if she registered.

And so Miranda entered my life. She is responsible for all the progress I have made. Each visit, we talk for 15 minutes - this is in itself such a lovely thing to do. We have got to know each other over the last year. I have laughed with her and cried with her - and pretty much everything in-between. She is someone who understands so much of what I am going through as she has seen it in other patients. After the chat comes the hard work! I have been given so many different exercises to help me. She has set me challenges - most of which I think I have completed. She has asked me what my next aim is and has provided me with exercises to help me get there. She has gone away to do research on some of my more peculiar symptoms - and not found an answer but she did try. As I am writing this, we are currently in Lockdown. A couple of weeks ago, she phoned to see how I was doing. We spoke for an hour. Even now, I smile when I remember the phone call. In a difficult time for all of us, the fact that she took so much time out of her day to talk to me makes me feel valued and happy.

The health insurance company never agreed to pay for Miranda. But she is worth every single penny we pay her. Thank you so much.

After about 11 weeks, I got an appointment thorough from the neuro physio department at The Alex. I went to the appointment, accompanied by my friend. I started off giving him my history - this took a little while. (Because although there were copious notes on my condition, they were at UHCW and hand written. Not on a computer with a file that could be shared between any interested parties...) We talked about what had happened, what I could do and what I would like to do. I told him I also had a neuro physio who was coming to the house to work with me. At the end of the session, he gave me some exercises to do and we made an appointment for two weeks time.

I arrived two weeks later, showing him how far I had got with my exercises. When he asked what the long scar was for on the side of my head, I nearly fell off the bed I was doing my exercises on. I appreciate that staff are busy, especially at a hospital. But I have to say, I would have hoped that he would have had a quick read of my notes before I arrived. Suffice to say, I didn't go back for another visit. And once more, I thanked my lucky stars that Miranda came to see me.

After 12 weeks, I had a letter from the Occupational Health Visitor and Home Visit Physiotherapist who were going to come to see me at home. I have to say, once again, that the NHS is great in a crisis, but…. If L had not been proactive and I had not been determined to improve what I could achieve, then I don't know what state I would have been in after 12 weeks. As it was, I could tell them that I was having some neuro physio at home, was now sleeping upstairs (as I had mastered being able to walk upstairs one stair at a time, and come down the same way), was able to cook a meal for myself and the family, could get in and out of the bath and various other things. They were happy that I had a good support network of friends and family to help me do the other jobs and that I didn't need any help from them. They left me an hour later happy that I was Ok and had their number to ring them if I needed anything. As I say, if I hadn't been in that position, I think a 3 month wait was perhaps a little too long.

I had a couple of appointments with Rehabilitation consultants during the nine months after my discharge. They were both very pleased with my progress. At the first appointment, I was given a top tip - to bring all my notes with me to each appointment so that anyone could have a quick glance at my history. This would stop me having to give edited highlights each time. At the second of these appointments, after I said I was starting a phased return to work in September, I was discharged.

In January, I waddled into my first post-op governance meeting. I managed to chair it - even if they did all have to listen very carefully whenever I talked - but it was great to see my fellow governors again, and the newly appointed head. The school has been a major part of my life for so long, it was wonderful to rejoin that community again. I have always felt that in governance, I have made a difference. As my mental faculties were still intact, I was able to resume this part of my life. Even if I did need a lift to and from the school…..

This brings me neatly on to driving. At my first post op meeting with Mr Beltechi, he said I would be able to drive after six months. After a lengthy conversation with a lovely man at the DVLA, he also confirmed that if a doctor had told me I was fit to drive, then this was OK. It took rather longer than six months for all the paperwork to come through. But after six months, I cautiously began driving again. The freedom…. It was absolutely wonderful.

In September, I began my phased return to work. I work as a Teaching Assistant with Year 4's. My work were wonderful throughout this whole process - and still are. I aim to be back full time in September 2020. I had a couple of occupational health meetings. At the first, we agreed that it was too soon but at the second, joy of joys, I would be allowed to start back at work for a few hours a week. The main concern was tiredness. In September, I was still sleeping for a couple of hours a day. I was also concerned that I would forget the many and frequent demands of the children on me.

In fact, I coped well with the frequent demands - using a trusted notebook. One of the main problems I found was projecting my voice across the classroom. The children who worked near me were great and would pass the message across the classroom. On several occasions, I was left in charge of the class. This was not a problem unless I needed to talk across them to get them all to be quiet. We had a handy button bell in our class and they quickly became used to the routine. If Mrs. Turnbull rings the bell, we all stop, look and listen.

On one memorable day, I was asked to look after the next door class of Year 4's. They were all chatting away and I wanted to give them the next instruction. So I rang the bell. And the whole class stood up and started to recite their times tables....! I frantically waved my arms about and got them to sit down and listen. And asked them what method the teacher used to get them to be quiet in their class!

Over the year, I have gradually increased my hours so that I aim to be working full time after a year. As I say, the people I work with - from the teachers in my class to my line-managers; from my fellow TA's to all the office staff and most especially to the children I work with who have taken their whispering, waddling TA completely in their stride, I thank you all. You make me smile each and every day.

I am finding, throughout my recovery, that I need to plan things far more than I have ever had to before. I will lie in bed planning what I am going to wear - or if I am going out in the evening, will spend many hours thinking about this. And on two occasions I have had complete meltdowns because I couldn't find what I wanted. Although there have been other things I could wear, it is the wasted mental time and space that I get cross about. We plan our meals and if they change at the last minute, especially without my knowledge, I find that very difficult. I plan journeys. I plan my day - down to hours. I plan routes I am going to drive. Everything I can think about ahead, I do. This has become slightly less essential as time goes on, but still happens.

One evening, we were going to go and sing for our choir MD's Mum's birthday. This was in a room in a pub - that we had been to before, but I remembered differently to how it is. We drove past the pub and I went into a complete (mental) tizzy. There were several steps going into the pub, lots of people there, and bouncers. So I was going to have to negotiate strange stairs, under the watchful eyes of two bouncers, and with lots of people around. Three things which I didn't like. And were not in my plan! I braved the stairs - on my own as L was parking the car - and got into the pub. There were lots of people around - it was very busy - and they didn't take much notice of the lady waddling through to the back with her stick. There was a bit of jostling, but I made it without falling over. While the whole incident was nerve-wracking, I did feel very pleased when I made it to the room at the back unscathed. I had coped with three things I didn't really feel comfortable doing and it had not been planned. Well done me.

Something we have always loved to do as a family is go camping. And this is something I very much wanted to return to doing. Our main holiday each year is two weeks camping in Cornwall. And before that, we usually go away for a couple of nights with our cycling friends in the Forest of Dean.

When I said I was going camping, I was generally greeted with a look of astonishment. Which turned to bemusement. Which ended up with an expression of shock. "Really? Are you sure that is wise?" "Are you mad?" "How are you going to manage?" And from Miranda "What do you need to achieve physically to be able to do that?"

So I spent several weeks practising standing up from the floor. And from low chairs.

And we were off. As it was only a couple of hours away, I knew that I could come home if I really needed to. But I thought it would all be under control.

When we arrived, I sat in a chair and L, H and J all had to put up the tent. This was a bit of a difference for the children as they usually met up with their friends and cycled around the campsite. The tent was put up and everything put in its place.

The physical aspect I found hardest was having to balance to get over the lip of the tent. This was achieved with a hand or a stick. So far so good. I had a concern that I wouldn't have enough warning to get to the toilet, as it was a significantly longer walk. In the weeks leading up to our trip away, I didn't think this would be so much of a problem. And I had planned on using some Tena Lady pads if I thought this would be a problem. Standing up inside the tent was no problem after the exercises I had carried out.

The biggest problem I had was not being in charge or even involved in the cooking/ washing up/ tent putting up or tent taking down. I sat in a chair watching all that was going on. While many may say this would be great, I found it very hard. I did manage to cook breakfast on the Sunday, but this was all. I found it very difficult to not be "doing my bit".

So in August we set off for our two week camping holiday in Cornwall. Although this was much further away, I knew I could come home if things really went badly. Once again, I was of very limited use in pitching the tent and setting up camp. H was a godsend - she knows how I like things to be set up so camp was pretty much how I wanted it to be.

We have made friends with a family who camp next to us so the children were off and happy. They had been told the news of our year so pretty much knew what to expect. On the other side, was another family that we had become friends with the previous year. I spent a little time trying to work out how to tell them what had happened. This is something I have got better at since then - diluting a very dramatic few months in hospital to a few sentences that are not too scary but convey quite what a journey it was.

One of the hardest things about our family holiday was wanting us to do all the things that we usually do; but realising that I was not physically able to do a lot of them or access quite a few places, and also recognising that I still needed to have a sleep regularly so sending them off to do things that I was less concerned about missing. I did still have the use of the wheelchair, so although I didn't like being in it all that much, my desire to join in with the family on the holiday outweighed my dislike of being pushed.

And I did take them all to Porthilly Bay which had been my special place that I went to as I went under anaesthetic. We took some lovely photos too.

In September, on the anniversary of my first scan, I decided to have a tea party. This was a small way to thank all of the people who had helped us, visited us, or in any way supported us over the last year. The guest list was initially all the people who had come up to visit me in UHCW with a few extra people added on.

In the run up to the party, I did wonder what I had decided to do. I had been back at work for a week by then and was feeling exhausted. But my friends and family, being as they are, were brilliant Lots of friends offered to bake cakes. A close friend and her family came for lunch beforehand (made by H of course) and helped transport the many boxes to the village hall. Another family came along to help set up the hall. And so many friends helped make the drinks and make sure all the food was put out as needed. The party wouldn't have flowed as well without them. Once again, thank you.

The party also turned out to be very therapeutic for me. I provided a few activities for people to have a think about. One is in Appendix B - what do these words mean? There was a "Guess what in the tissue box" game. I had my playlist on in the background. There were pictures of my pureed meals for people to guess at. And a box full of sweets (I had been sent this as a gift while I was in hospital and it proved very popular both with my family and with visiting children of my hospital friends.) It was great being able to chat to so many friends and important people to me. I am only sorry that I didn't get the chance to speak to you all.

After the party, I found I was thinking a lot less about my time in hospital.

So the last part of 2019 to write about, and the most tricky, is how I felt about things as the year went on.

Frustration, irritation and guilt are three emotions that run strongly through the year. As I say, I was always very black and white about the operation - I would live or die. I hadn't really prepared myself for an in-between; but that is where I found myself.

When talking to a friend the other day, she reminded me that when she visited me in hospital, I would frequently say "I don't mind if I am in a wheelchair for the rest of my life. At least I have a rest of my life." While I am still so very grateful to be here, the year has not been without challenges.

Between January and March, I was at home, not able to go anywhere. I was reliant on friends coming to visit me - which they did. But on days when I had no-one, I would feel very sorry for myself. I was able to get up from the sofa, go to the toilet, make myself a bowl of soup for lunch and other mundane tasks. But I still needed people to get the children to and from school, to take them to clubs, to do most of the cooking (this fell to H), to do the cleaning, to get me and the children to any appointments that they had. All my life, I have been the one to do this for other people. That is who I am. And I found it so very, very difficult to accept help from other people - be they family or friends (or even, in one case, a complete stranger!) I was also still having to sleep for a large chunk of every day (approximately 120 minutes). As I was not confident going up the stairs, I would sleep on the sofa under a blanket. The sofa is not quite the same as it was at the start of 2019...... I would have boxes set up near the sofa with everything I might need; books, craft things, notebooks, pens, my diary, snacks, headphones, a charging cable... they became a larger (and immovable) Tesco Value Tissue box. My life was in them.

In April, I was slowly and cautiously driving again. I was able to go and collect J from school. The look on his face the first time I picked him up is something that will stay with me forever. It makes me smile every time I think of it. Although I collected him, we stayed with the same routine for taking the children to school.

This was partly because of something that I have been left with since the operation. Tri-geminal Nerualgia. There is a nerve that enters the face by the temple. It then splits into three with one part going to the forehead, one to just under the eye and the third to the bottom of the face. Pretty much every morning, I get an attack of neuralgia, down the left side of my face, when my head goes vertical. Is it a result of my brain moving around as there is now a gap for it to move into? Is it a result of nerves in my brain being very irritated? The health professionals don't know. I don't know. But I do know that this is the most painful condition I have ever suffered from. The pain has made me cry - frequently - and I often sit there trying to hold my head together. On a couple of occasions, the pain has been so bad that I have literally tried to pull my face off. Attacks last anywhere from 30 to 150 minutes. During that time, I have what is called scrunchies (which feel like someone has put hot foil on my face and is scrunching it up) and stabbies (which feel like someone is driving a hot nail into my head). As well as having an attack in the morning, I also tend to have one in the afternoon too - at a time to be decided upon by my nerves! I have also been woken up in the night with an attack, and had them as I am trying to go to sleep. There seems to be no pattern to them, and nothing specific that sets them off. I am taking gabapentin and tegretol - both neuro specific painkillers - which can diminish the length and severity of the attacks. But after a few months, I am back to the GP asking her to increase the dose.

Over the year, I found it difficult to be so reliant on the family. I was a stay-at-home Mum for years, and then I worked part time so still did the majority of the household chores and childcare. Doing tasks that I hadn't thought required any effort, were now things that I found hard to do. H did most of the cooking. I managed to cook a few meals but found them totally exhausting. Even getting something out of a top cupboard produced yelps of pain (my left shoulder is very hard to move). I never knew how much I would miss doing my washing. It was about October before I managed to take my clean washing upstairs. And about December before I managed a way to take the dirty washing downstairs. And putting away my clean clothes? Don't worry - I have been wearing clean clothes. L does the washing every weekend - or as needed.

Towards the end of the year, I have had the strength and balance to do some hoovering. I can clean the downstairs cloakroom. I can wipe down all the surfaces in the kitchen. Stacking and unstacking the dishwasher was something I could do some days and not others. Bending down repeatedly made me very dizzy. I could walk upstairs "normally" (one foot on each step rather than having to put one foot on a step and follow it by the other foot on the same step). I was walking around outside without a stick - although I did use an arm or other support if I was walking up or down a slope).

So, some of the not so good things about 2019? Anyone who has had a stroke or other brain injury will tell you about the fatigue. It is absolute. It can come out of nowhere - it is like hitting a wall and once you have hit it, you just have to have a nap or go to bed. Every day I needed a nap.

And the frustration at not being the person I was. I was now reliant on friends and family for so much. And although I know they don't mind - L will say (rightly) that I would do the same for anyone in the family - I still don't like it. Before my operation, I was the one that did things for others. I find it very difficult now the shoe is on the other foot. And the fatigue….

And each time I have gone to the hospital to get the results of my scan, I feel so scared. My head tells me that nothing that bad could have grown in 6 months. But my heart? It tells a different story. And the fatigue…..

And the hardest thing for me during 2019 was trying to adapt to my new place in the family. I was always the go-to person in the family. And suddenly I wasn't. I think this was partly to protect me but also because for the hardest 3 months in our family's life, I not only wasn't there to help out, I was the cause. Some of this change was a good thing. L did far more in the house than he used to, but so did the children - particularly H. At a time when she was studying for her GCSE's, she was also caring for me physically and looking after the house. J does lots of little jobs for me - ones that I can do but know I will have more energy later if I don't.

Both children do their own washing - from collecting off the floor (!) to putting it in the washing machine, drying it, ironing it if needed and putting it away. Or should I say both children can do all that... it does require a little nagging though! Especially the putting away part of the job! So I am still good at the nagging part. Although they have to be downstairs as my voice doesn't carry upstairs.

Doing the supermarket shopping is something else that used to be my domain and is now not. L is fantastic at getting a list and buying all the things on it. Nothing more and nothing less. I have to agree that the cost of a weekly shop has gone down somewhat without my impulse buys - from the middle aisles in Aldi! And we needed to have a complete list of what was needed. Which can be difficult when you are not doing most of the cooking.....The tiredness I feel when cooking one meal for four people is more than I ever thought would be possible..

Weekends were a time which I found particularly hard. Although it was great having the family around, it was also a time when I felt really guilty. They would spend their weekends rushing around doing jobs and I couldn't help, Not only that, I couldn't do the jobs while I was at home during the week. And not only that, I contributed to the number of jobs that needed doing. It was so tiring having them all around. It is amazing to me how tiring interacting with other people is. There was very little quiet time when I could just be alone with my thoughts - and let my brain have a rest. And have I mentioned the fatigue??

But it's not all doom and gloom. L and I had wanted to take the children to New Zealand for years. But the cost was more than we could reasonably save.

In April, L was told that his job would be made redundant. There followed a lot of discussions where it was realised by us that they still wanted him at the company but in a different role, with a new boss. It was all very complicated but one option given to him was to take a redundancy payout. We decided that this was the best option for us and he got himself a new job straight away. So win-win for us. And we now had enough money to take us all to New Zealand.

I then spent many hours of 2019 looking at flights, accommodation and what we would do when we got there. We were planning to go for two weeks in April 2021. This was to be a lovely treat for the family after a tough 18 months.

I realised that I was important to a far wider group of people than I could ever have imagined. I had cards, notes, emails and visits from all sorts of people telling me what an impact (positive!) I had had on a part of their lives. This really helped me to feel good about myself at a time when that was not an easy thing to do.

And I was slowly, but oh so surely, getting more mobility and feeling better about things.. I was able to get out and about with friends and family - all be it not quite as quickly as before. A friend and I went to visit another friend in their caravan. We had talked about this trip a lot whilst I was in hospital. It felt so good for it to be finally happening. By the end of the year, I was back doing everything that I was doing pre September 2018. A bit more slowly perhaps, but managing to do it all. And both Di and Miranda said I was doing more than many people would do without having a brain tumour and having had a stroke. And we went away for Christmas. And had the neighbours round for pre-Christmas drinks. Again, although these were tiring, it was great to be doing normal things.

The biggest plus for me in 2019 was getting back to work. I needed to stop sitting around at home for my mental health. I felt I could be of use to the children I worked with, so that is where I wanted to be. Miranda thought that physically, I was not quite ready, but on balance, for the whole me, it was something that needed to happen And it made me feel sooo good. Interacting with other adults as well as the children was just the tonic I needed to boost my recovery further.

And the fatigue... Although over the year, the amount I needed to sleep did drop. By the end of the year, I didn't need to sleep every day. But if I missed a day, I would have a massive nap the next day. It was good to know that I could go for a day without sleeping. Because otherwise, my days were taken up with doing a school run, coming home and doing something (usually watching something on iPlayer), having some lunch - on a good day - and sleeping before going to do the school run again. This meant I had little time to do much else. But as L said, this is what a typical day at work is like for him - with just the weekends to do things.

PART 3

2020 - Year of Acceptannce

I am writing this during Lockdown. This has been an odd time for all of us. Although my 3 months at home, before I could go out on my own, has strangely prepared me for this, back then, however, I could have visitors and I didn't have children at home all the time.

And of course, we didn't make it to New Zealand. On the plus side, we aim to go in April 2021 - and all the planning is done!

A lot of my time with Di was spent trying to accept the new me. I realised I couldn't do this until I knew what the new me was going to be. So over lockdown, I have stopped doing my physio. I will start doing it again, but only once I am happy with the person I am now. Lucinda 2.0. Then I can pick up from where I left off, and make more progress. Perhaps Lucinda 2.1 will be "released". And who knows which editions after that?

Writing my story has taken many hours of thought. I have committed to paper things that I remembered from hospital that I had rarely thought about and things that I spent a lot of time thinking about. In this way, it has helped me put my experience to bed. It will always be something that happened to me, but I need to reframe my life.

In talking to the family over the last two months, it has become clear to me that my life consists of pre and post op. Theirs doesn't. The experience for them was something that no one should have to go through but was not life-changing. This made me feel very upset. Why has something that turned my life upside down not turned theirs upside down either? I don't know the answer to that but I know that I am more understanding of their view point now.

I am still struggling to find my place in the family. But I am accepting that it has changed. And we probably have a far more balanced family life than we did. And that has got to be a good thing. (I am not sure L would agree in the more chaotic moments!) When I really think about it, there is a lot that I can and do contribute. It is just not as much and is different.

And even the emotional support is now often not my job. Frequently, when they used to come to talk to me or shout for me, it is now L that they call for. And that hurts more than the children will ever know (until now!) But I have to reconcile in my head that the most important thing is that they are still asking for help -

most of the time. Their mental well-being is paramount, and whoever they get support from, at least they are getting it. My feelings need to come second on this one.

I have been encouraged to put my needs higher up the pecking order of my life. This is something that I have never really done. If a friend or family member needed something, I would always do it - even if it put me out to do so. I am trying very hard not to do this now. If someone asks me to do a job, I will try to count to 10 before agreeing. And I have even been known to say no sometimes! If I am to improve more physically, my physio needs to happen, regardless of what else is happening in the house. For me to stay healthy mentally, I need to take some time to look out at my beautiful garden (without looking at all the little jobs that I feel guilty that I should be able to do but can't).

And I don't feel nearly as guilty about the events of the last year and a half as I used to. I accept that I didn't cause any of this, nor is there anything I could have done to prevent it happening. Although my family's life has changed, they would all far rather I was in it and they had to do extra chores, than not in it. I think I will always feel some amount of guilt that they all have to do more work and I can do far less than I used to , but that is just me. And I am feeling better about things.

Physically, I am not where I was before this story began, and I am not where I would like to be. I would like to be able to walk downstairs "normally" and be able to be completely independent. I would like to be able to cook a meal without feeling exhausted, to be able to go for walks in fields and to be able to carry my washing up and down stairs. But when I think of where I have come from, I feel proud of myself.

I was challenged by Miranda to do a 5km run/walk in 2020. So I signed myself up for The Stroke Association run in March. I received lots of sponsorship. And the run was cancelled due to the Covid-19 outbreak. But I am still aiming to do it - by joining in one of our local Park Runs - with H as my support.   So watch this space....

In writing this story, there is something that all readers should be aware of. Other than a bit (or a big bit) of a waddle when I walk, I look pretty normal from the outside.   However, the effort that goes into every bit of every day should not be underestimated.

If you turn up to work with wet hair, people would think you have had a shower before coming out to work (if they even noticed). For me to have a shower requires quite gargantuan effort. It is absolutely exhausting. And that is before I have even started my day.

There is a theory I have found that I identify with - The Spoon Theory. It talks about people having a certain number of blocks of energy (spoons) to use in a day. And once you have used all your spoons, you have no choice but to rest up until you make some more spoons. Dressing requires a spoon. Showering requires a spoon - maybe two if you are washing your hair. Walking downstairs is definitely a spoon for me…. And so it goes on. For people who have had strokes or other brain injuries, fatigue and managing fatigue is a fact of life. I have a friend who had a stroke over 10 years ago. She still has to factor a nap into each and every day.

So if you see me, be patient. The tiredness can show as extra wobbly walking, my brain working more slowly than usual (I often forget words - particularly names and places), my speech slurring (my still-wonky tongue is less and less obedient, the more tired I get) or even a reluctance to do small tasks (each task might require a spoon and I might be trying to make another spoon or save a spoon for a later activity).

So here is the story of Lucinda 2.0 But I am confident that there will be a 2.1 at some point soon. But if there isn't? Life is pretty good as it is. And as I said in hospital, at least I have a life to live.

Postscript – or Lucinda 2.1

I am now coming up to six years after the story began. Whilst rereading the story, and particularly the odd things my body did or didn't do, I am struck by how much of that has not changed. My life is still governed by trigeminal neuralgia and neuro fatigue. The neuralgia seems to be brought on by vibrations – particularly through my feet. This means that I am not walking very much. As a result, I am losing a lot of my core strength, so when I do walk I am very wobbly!

I still come in from work and have a sleep, although not for as long. And I can go for a few days without a nap. But I do pay for it.

And I still only cry from one eye.

On a recent visit to A and E, it was very much brought home how much the discovery of my tumour, and the repercussions of it, had on my family. With any accident or incident, there is a very real and huge worry that the tumour is recurring (as we know it will one day). Although I know there is nothing I did to cause the tumour, knowing how much it still affects the family, six years on, is very difficult and fills me with feelings of guilt.

However, I go away with my family and, thanks to a great scooter, can enjoy walks with them and spending time doing the things we used to do.

I am still working part time at my school. They are very supportive and accommodating to my needs. It is great to be somewhere where at least a few people know the old me as well as the new one. However much I am getting used to the new me, I have realized that it is incredibly important to me that some people remember the old me and all that I was capable of then.

Due to my paralysed vocal cord (the botox is wearing off and it doesn't work nearly as well now), I find social situations very difficult. I cannot project my voice so can't be heard over lots of background noise. This can prove interesting in class. But with the help of some fantastic and completely accepting children, I get by.

I am talking to another therapist. The focus this time is on helping me to accept who I am now and giving me confidence to believe in that person. It may take a while, but I think progress is being made.

BOOK TITLE

I am also living a life where I need care. This is mainly given by my daughter, but she is very ably supported by L and J. I find it very difficult to not only be able to help out with jobs round the house but also to be contributing to them. This situation results in a lot of frustration on all our parts.

But, all in all, life is good. Where problems arise, solutions are found. I am managing to do more of the things that I want to be able to do thanks to the ever present support of family and friends. You only realise how lucky you are when life throws you a lemon and they all help you make lemonade.

Each moment of life is precious. Enjoy it

APPENDIX A

Playlist – Counting Sheep in Coventry

These songs made it on to my playlist for a variety of reasons: they were easy to sing, they brought back a good memory, they were sung by the choir I sing in-Notorious (this meant I was instantly taken back to a concert venue and I knew all the words - yes - OBH, Clare) or they had a certain meaning for me whilst in hospital.

All of these reasons meant I was distracted from the thoughts flying round my brain while Counting Sheep in Coventry.

Song	Artist	Reason
Baby, I love your way	Big Mountain	One I like and can sing along to
Ben	Michael Jackson	Again, one I can sing along to
Bills	LunchMoney Lewis	Fabulous memories of (trying) to sing along to this with 6 children in the car on a great weekend away with friends
Calling Occupants of Interplanetary Craft	Carpenters	A great song sung by Notorious. Instantly standing in the Electric Cinema in Birmingham
Chilli Con Carne	Real Group	Another Notorious song. This time I am standing in The Prince of Wales, Moseley
Crazy Crazy Nights	Kiss	And this time, I am in Kings Heath Cricket Club
Here Comes the Sun	The Beatles	And now I am in Christ Church, Selly Park
I Get a Kick Out of You	Frank Sinatra	And now I am in The Kings Head, Bearwood
I Saw Her Standing There	The Beatles	This time I am in the school hall learning a dance to teach the children for the fete
I Wanne Be the Only One	Eternal	This one is just one I like singing along to.
Ill Wind	Flanders and	One I know all the words to - and it still makes me

	Swann	smile
Isn't She Lovely	Stevie Wonder	One I can sing along to
No More "I love you"'s	Annie Lennox	Back to The Cricket Club in Kings Heath
Survival	Muse	And still in The Cricket Club
Air Guitar	McBusted	Another one I like to sing along to (don't judge me too harshly...)
History	One Direction	This was sung by son's class as their leavers song - with some adapted words. So I am sitting in his old school hall.
The Land of Make Believe	Bucks Fizz	This one takes me back to my old kitchen, singing along to this with my Mum while she cooked dinner
Let the River Run	Carly Simon	Back to Notorious. This time we are in a cave in Dudley....
Los Olivados	Flanders and Swann	This one is not a song but one of their stories. And I love it and hear a new detail each time.
evolting Children	From Matilda the Musical	A great musical with some fantastic songs to sing along to.
Santa Baby	Ella Fitzgerald	This version that I remember is in The Midlands Arts Centre (The MAC)
Slow Train	Flanders and Swann	A beautiful song. I like remembering the song when I see somewhere that is mentioned in it

We Will Rock You	Queen	Now I am actually rehearsing for this in the MAC before the concert
When I Grow Up	From Matilda	I love the words to this song - so apt
99 Red Balloons	Nena	This reminds of singing along in the car with the children. We are just arriving at a shopping centre in
White Wine in the Sun	Tim Minchin	This concert was in The Dark Horse
Thank You for Being a Friend	Andrew Gold	The words are so apt for all my wonderful friends
That's What Friends Are For	Dionne Warwick	The same as above
I'm Still Standing	Elton John	Sung by me whenever I managed to stand unaided and then be "Still Standing" It was usually accompanied by a big grin!
Ring My Bell	Anita Ward	Often sung by me in the night when the ringing of the bell went unanswered. This was a good distraction from the fact that I (usually) needed the loo...
I'm Here	From Matilda	Although this song is called I'm Here, a recurring line in the song is "Don't Cry". I sang this to myself frequently to try to stop myself crying - either before or during the event.
Friends Theme Tune	Sung by Notorious	This was what was sung for me by my friends in the fabulous Notorious choir
What a Difference a	Dinah	Again, a song that frequently went round my head when I would wake up feeling so much better than

Day Makes	Washington	the day before (and sometimes when I was feeling so much worse too!)
The Long and Winding Road	The Beatles	This song sums up my ongoing journey
The Sloth	Flanders and Swann	What a great little song - and I love sloths!
The Ostrich	Flanders and Swann	This song reminds me of going into a car park in Maidstone - if you want more detail, you will need to listen to the song and then ask me!
Rock the Boat	The Hues Corporation	This time I am in the canal boat taking us back from our concert in Dudley Caves
Making Your Mind Up	Bucks Fizz	I am now dancing round the kitchen with my Mum many years ago. She is frying onions…. Yum
School Song	From Matilda	I am always trying to remember the words to this one. Still trying……

APPENDIX B

How much attention were you paying?

Whilst in hospital, many new words entered my vocabulary. The following words are all mentioned - and described - in the story. Can you match the word with the meaning?

(Warning: do not do this if you are squeamish)

Word	Meaning
Choughy	A daily injection to help stop blood clotting
Lactulose	The description of a wound that is pussy with skin coming off
Clexane	A condition that affects speech, swallowing , coordination, balance, and writing among other things.
Aspirate	A type of brain tumour - usually grade 1
Ataxia	Something given to you to help loosen stools
Meningioma	A scale used to describe how loose a stool is
Bristol Stool Scale	The liquid contents of the stomach

APPENDIX C

Lucinda 2.0

Below is a list of the most obvious things to me that are different post op. Some of these are as a result of the stroke, some as a result of ataxia - and some appear to be just me.....

- I have no feelings of pain in the right side of my body
- I cannot detect temperature in the right side of my body
- The inside of my left nostril is constantly inflamed. And bleeds frequently.
- I have very little sense of smell.
- I can walk upstairs normally - with the help of a rail

- I am starting to walk downstairs normally - with the help of two rails.
- I have no libido
- I need to sleep for an hour a day at least
- I can stand for the time it takes to cook a family meal - but it exhausts me.
- I have debilitating neuralgia. I have an attack every morning and usually one every afternoon too. When out walking, I usually have an attack too.
- My tongue goes to the left. It makes things hard to clear from the right side of my mouth.
- The bottom left quarter of my skull feels very odd.
- I can't lift my left arm above my head
- I can't project my voice - in a classroom or on a zoom call.
- I have a very peculiar sneeze!
- I have a constant tension headache - from the pain or anticipation thereof.
- I am less able to multitask
- When I cry (which is every day..), I only shed tears from my right eye.
- And if I exert pressure on any part of my body (such as opening the front door, turning a tap on or off), I get shooting pains down the left side of my head

So there you have it. The odd little world I live in!

APPENDIX D

Thank yous

I cannot begin to list everyone whom I need to thank. If you are not on this list, it is not because you do not deserve thanks but because I can't remember your name - just your face (this is a common problem I have post op). So in no particular order:

First and foremost, my fantastic family. So many of you came to visit me, sent me cards or emails, phoned me, looked after the immediate family - the list goes on. So thanks to

L, H, J, AG, CG, DG, AT, MT, GT, IT, JT, RT

And all who looked after me at UHCW and the Alex Hospital from the consultants through to the cleaning staff. Between you, you all saved my life - from literally removing my tumour to smiling and chatting to me whilst cleaning under the bed.

So in no particular order:

Mr Beltechi and his team; Ioan, Martin, Hollie, Kylie, the physios, the occupational health team - I can only remember Chris' name, Marichelle, all the cheerful porters (I didn't meet any who weren't cheerful), the cleaning staff, the HCAs, the dieticians, the psychologists, the SALT team, plastic surgeons and all the staff in Radiology.

And of course Dr Birling and Dr Ash at my local GP practice who first guessed something was not quite right and then have helped me through the last eighteen months.

And the medical professionals who have helped me since I have come home - speech therapists, occupational therapists, physiotherapists and rehabilitation specialists.

And thank yous also need to go to Di, Lisa and Miranda.

And where do I begin with the long, long list of friends who have been there for me and the family? You have visited, emailed, phoned, ferried me (and my children) round the West Midlands, taken me to hospital appointments, taken me to GP appointments, taken my children to hospital appointments and been a general source of support for me. This would have been a very different story without you...

So again, in no particular order:

BL, ML, TH, SH, AH, LH, SD, SB, JB, JB, DB, EH, CH, AH, SH, LY, LJ, MW, RN, EB, TH, TB, AS, AMR and all my friends at OLMC, RH, DH, AL, SM, RH, RA, AR, SJ, RJ. GJ, KJ, LJ, BT, SP, EP, WH, KD, KB, PB, NB, AO, CO, DS, RW, PY, TM, TD, KS, JD, JC,JR CC, AM, ST, AC, KD, JB, RM, SP, ED, CE and all my 'Notorious' friends, SM, SM.

And below are the lyrics to two songs that begin to sum up how I feel about my friends.

That's What Friends Are For

Dionne Warwick

And I never thought I'd feel this way
And as far as I'm concerned
I'm glad I got the chance to say
That I do believe, I love you

And if I should ever go away
Well, then close your eyes and try
To feel the way we do today
And then if you can remember

Keep smiling, keep shining
Knowing you can always count on me, for sure
That's what friends are for
For good times and bad times
I'll be on your side forever more
That's what friends are for

Well, you came in loving me
And now there's so much more I see
And so by the way
I thank you

Oh and then for the times when we're apart
Well, then close your eyes and know
The words are coming from my heart
And then if you can remember

Keep smiling and keep shining
Knowing you can always count on me, for sure
That's what friends are for
In good times and bad times
I'll be on your side forever more
That's what friends are for

Thank You for Being a Friend

Andrew Gold

Thank you for being a friend
Traveled down a road and back again
Your heart is true, you're a pal and a confidantI'm
not ashamed to say
I hope it always will stay this way
My hat is off, won't you stand up and take a bow

And if you threw a party
Invited everyone you knew
Well, you would see the biggest gift would be from
me
And the card attached would say

Thank you for being a friend
Thank you for being a friend
Thank you for being a friend
Thank you for being a friend

If it's a car you lack
I'd surely buy you a Cadillac
Whatever you need any time of the day or night

I'm not ashamed to say
I hope it always will stay this way
My hat is off, won't you stand up and take a bow

And when we both get older
With walking canes and hair of gray
Have no fear even though it's hard to hear
I will stand here close and say

Thank you for being a friend (I wanna thank you)
Thank you for being a friend (I wanna thank you)
Thank you for being a friend (I wanna thank you)
Thank you for being a friend (I wanna thank
you)Let me tell you about a friend (I wanna thank
you)
Thank you for being a friend (I wanna thank you)
Thank you for being a friend (I wanna thank you)
Thank you for being a friend (I wanna thank you)

And when we die and float away
Into the night the Milky Way
You'll hear me call as we ascend
I'll say your name then once again

Thank you for being a

Thank you for being a friend (I want to thank you)

ABOUT THE AUTHOR

Lucinda lives in England with her family. Three years on, she is still working, enjoying spending time with her family – and crying out of only one eye!!

Printed in Great Britain
by Amazon

43212877R00069